The Vibrant Guide to Mediterranean Diet

A Complete Collection of Appetizing Recipes to Eat the
Mediterranean Way

America Best Recipes

Table of contents

3

4

Easy Seafood French Stew

Preparation Time: 10 minutes

Cooking Time: 45 minutes

Servings: 12

Ingredients:

- Pepper and Salt
- 1/2 lb. littleneck clams
- 1/2 lb. mussels
- 1 lb. shrimp, peeled and deveined
- 1 large lobster
- 2 lbs. assorted small whole fresh fish, scaled and cleaned
- 2 tbsp. parsley, finely chopped
- 2 tbsp. garlic, chopped
- 1 cup fennel, julienned
- Juice and zest of one orange
- 3 cups tomatoes, peeled, seeded, and chopped
- 1 cup leeks, julienned
- Pinch of Saffron

Stew Ingredients:

- 1 cup white wine
- Water
- 1 lb. fish bones
- 2 sprigs thyme
- 8 peppercorns
- 1 bay leaf
- 3 cloves garlic
- Salt and pepper
- 1/2 cup chopped celery
- 1/2 cup chopped onion
- 2 tbsp. olive oil

Directions:

1. Do the stew: Heat oil in a large saucepan. Sauté the celery and onions for 3 minutes. Season with pepper and salt. Stir in the garlic and cook for about a minute. Add the thyme, peppercorns, and bay leaves. Stir in the wine, water and fish bones. Let it boil then before reducing to a simmer. Take the pan off the fire and strain broth into another container.

2. For the Bouillabaisse: Bring the strained broth to a simmer and stir in the parsley, leeks, orange juice, orange zest, garlic, fennel, tomatoes and saffron. Sprinkle with pepper and salt. Stir in the lobsters and fish. Let it simmer for eight minutes before stirring in the clams, mussels and shrimps. For six minutes, allow to cook while covered before seasoning again with pepper and salt.

3. Assemble in a shallow dish all the seafood and pour the broth over it.

Nutrition:

Calories: 348;

Carbs: 20.0g;

Protein: 31.8g;

Fat: 15.2g

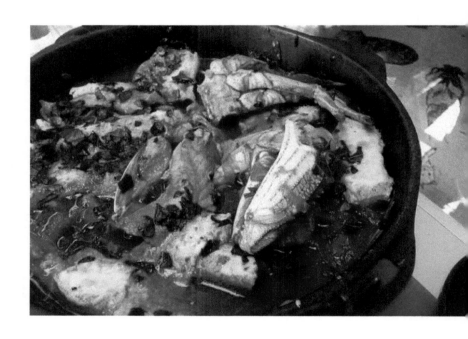

Fresh and No-Cook Oysters

Preparation Time: 10 minutes

Cooking Time: 5 minutes

Servings: 4

Ingredients:

- 2 lemons
- 24 medium oysters
- tabasco sauce

Directions:

1. If you are a newbie when it comes to eating oysters, then I suggest that you blanch the oysters before eating.

2. For some, eating oysters raw is a great way to enjoy this dish because of the consistency and juiciness of raw oysters. Plus, adding lemon juice prior to eating the raw oysters cooks it a bit.

3. So, to blanch oysters, bring a big pot of water to a rolling boil. Add oysters in batches of 6-10 pieces. Leave on boiling pot of water between 3-5 minutes and remove oysters right away. To eat oysters, squeeze lemon juice on oyster on shell, add tabasco as desired and eat.

Nutrition:

Calories: 247;

Protein: 29g;

Fat: 7g;

Carbs: 17g

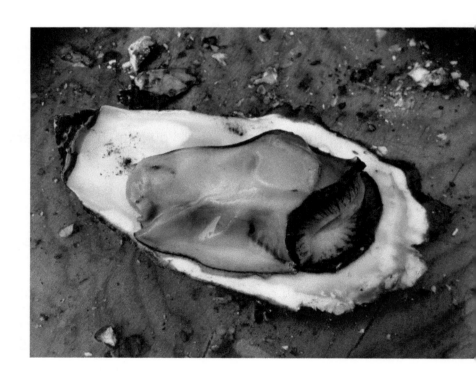

Easy Broiled Lobster Tails

Preparation Time: 10 minutes

Cooking Time: 10 minutes

Servings: 2

Ingredients:

- 1 6-oz frozen lobster tails
- 1 tbsp. olive oil
- 1 tsp. lemon pepper seasoning

Directions:

4. Preheat oven broiler.
5. With kitchen scissors, cut thawed lobster tails in half lengthwise.
6. Brush with oil the exposed lobster meat. Season with lemon pepper.
7. Place lobster tails in baking sheet with exposed meat facing up.
8. Place on top broiler rack and broil for 10 minutes until lobster meat is lightly browned on the sides and center meat is opaque. Serve and enjoy.

Nutrition: Calories: 175.6; Protein: 23g; Fat: 10g; Carbs: 18.4g

Ginger Scallion Sauce over Seared Ahi

Preparation Time: 10 minutes

Cooking Time: 6 minutes

Servings: 4

Ingredients:

- 1 bunch scallions, bottoms removed, finely chopped
- 1 tbsp. rice wine vinegar
- 1 tbsp.. Bragg's liquid amino
- 16-oz ahi tuna steaks
- 2 tbsp.. fresh ginger, peeled and grated
- 3 tbsp.. coconut oil, melted
- Pepper and salt to taste

Directions:

1. In a small bowl mix together vinegar, 2 tbsp.. oil soy sauce, ginger and scallions. Put aside.
2. On medium fire, place a large saucepan and heat remaining oil. Once oil is hot and starts to smoke, sear tuna until deeply browned or for two minutes per side.
3. Place seared tuna on a serving platter and let it stand for 5 minutes before slicing into 1-inch thick strips.
4. Drizzle ginger-scallion mixture over seared tuna, serve and enjoy.

Nutrition:

Calories: 247;

Protein: 29g;

Fat: 1g;

Carbs: 8g

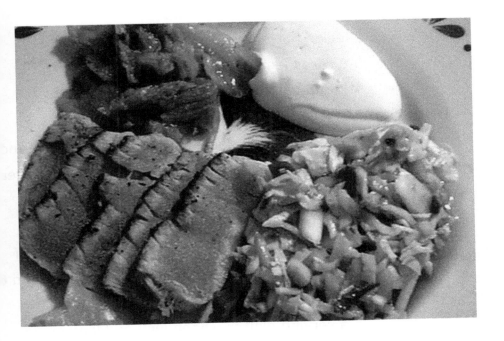

Healthy Poached Trout

Preparation Time: 10 minutes

Cooking Time: 10 minutes

Servings: 2

Ingredients:

- 1 8-oz boneless, skin on trout fillet
- 2 cups chicken broth or water
- 2 leeks, halved
- 6-8 slices lemon
- salt and pepper to taste

Directions:

1. On medium fire, place a large nonstick skillet an arrange leeks and lemons on pan in a layer. Cove with soup stock or water and bring to a simmer.
2. Meanwhile, season trout on both sides with pepper and salt. Place trout on simmering pan of water. Cover and cook until trout is flaky, around minutes.
3. In a serving platter, spoon leek and lemons on bottom of plate, top with trout and spoon sauce into plate. Serve and enjoy.

Nutrition:

Calories: 360.2;

Protein: 13.8g;

Fat: 7.5g;

Carbs: 51.5g

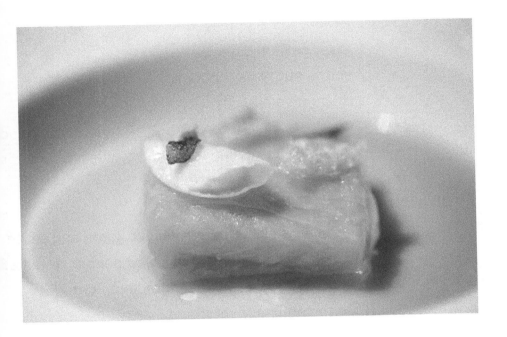

Leftover Salmon Salad Power Bowls

Preparation Time: 10 minutes

Cooking Time: 10 minutes

Servings: 1

Ingredients:

- ½ cup raspberries
- ½ cup zucchini, sliced
- 1 lemon, juice squeezed
- 1 tbsp. balsamic glaze
- 2 sprigs of thyme, chopped
- 2 tbsp. olive oil
- 4 cups seasonal greens
- 4 oz. leftover grilled salmon
- Salt and pepper to taste

Directions:

1. Heat oil in a skillet over medium flame and sauté the zucchini. Season with salt and pepper to taste
2. In a mixing bowl, mix all ingredients together.
3. Toss to combine everything.
4. Sprinkle with nut cheese.

Nutrition:

Calories: 450.3;

Fat: 35.5 g;

Protein: 23.4g;

Carbs: 9.3 g

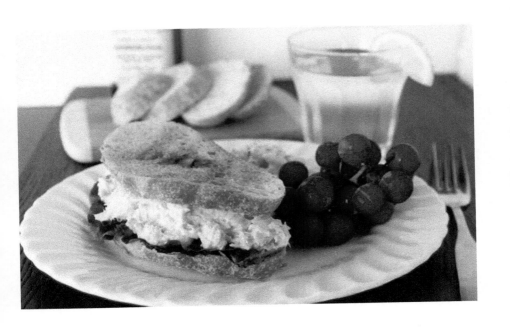

Lemon-Garlic Baked Halibut

Preparation Time: 10 minutes

Cooking Time: 15 minutes

Servings: 2

Ingredients:

- 1 large garlic clove, minced
- 1 tbsp. chopped flat leaf parsley
- 1 tsp. olive oil
- 2 5-oz boneless, skin-on halibut fillets
- 2 tsp. lemon zest
- Juice of ½ lemon, divided
- Salt and pepper to taste

Directions:

1. Grease a baking dish with cooking spray and preheat oven to 400oF.

2. Place halibut with skin touching the dish and drizzle with olive oil.
3. Season with pepper and salt.
4. Pop into the oven and bake until flaky around 12-15 minutes.
5. Remove from oven and drizzle with remaining lemon juice, serve and enjoy with a side of salad greens.

Nutrition:

Calories: 315.3;

Protein: 14.1g;

Fat: 10.5g;

Carbs: 36.6g

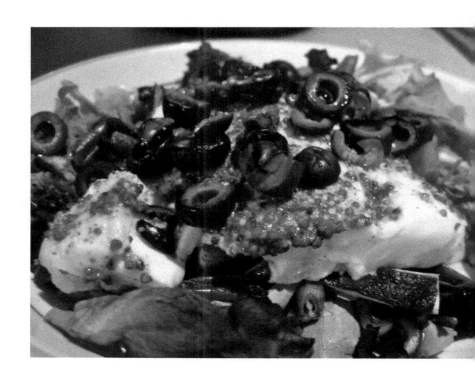

Minty-Cucumber Yogurt Topped Grilled Fish

Preparation Time: 10 minutes

Cooking Time: 2 minutes

Servings: 4

Ingredients:

- ¼ cup 2% plain Greek yogurt
- ¼ tsp. + 1/8 tsp. salt
- ¼ tsp. black pepper
- ½ green onion, finely chopped
- ½ tsp. dried oregano
- 1 tbsp. finely chopped fresh mint leaves
- 3 tbsp. finely chopped English cucumber
- 4 5-oz cod fillets
- Cooking oil as needed

Directions:

1. Brush grill grate with oil and preheat grill to high.
2. Season cod fillets on both sides with pepper, ¼ tsp. salt and oregano.
3. Grill cod for 3 minutes per side or until cooked to desired doneness.
4. Mix thoroughly 1/8 tsp. salt, onion, mint, cucumber and yogurt in a small bowl. Serve cod with a dollop of the dressing. This dish can be paired with salad greens or brown rice.

Nutrition:

Calories: 253.5;

Protein: 25.5g;

Fat: 1g;

Carbs: 5g

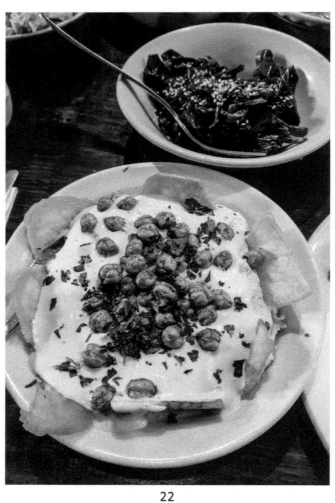

One-Pot Seafood Chowder

Preparation Time: 10 minutes

Cooking Time: 10 minutes

Servings: 3

Ingredients:

- 3 cans coconut milk
- 1 tbsp. garlic, minced
- Salt and pepper to taste
- 3 cans clams, chopped
- 2 cans shrimps, canned
- 1 package fresh shrimps, shelled and deveined
- 1 can corn, drained
- 4 large potatoes, diced
- 2 carrots, peeled and chopped
- 2 celery stalks, chopped

Directions:

1. Place all ingredients in a pot and give a good stir to mix everything.
2. Close the lid and turn on the heat to medium.
3. Bring to a boil and allow to simmer for 10 minutes.
4. Place in individual containers.
5. Put a label and store in the fridge.
6. Allow to warm at room temperature before heating in the microwave oven.

Nutrition:

Calories: 532;

Carbs: 92.5g;

Protein: 25.3g;

Fat: 6.7g

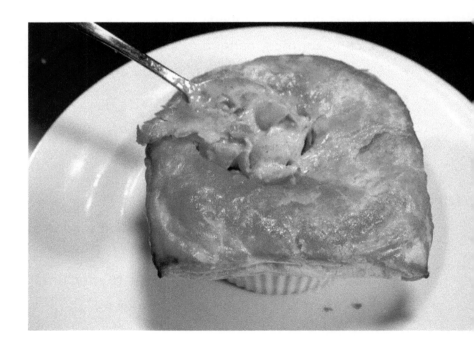

Orange Rosemary Seared Salmon

Preparation Time: 10 minutes

Cooking Time: 10 minutes

Servings: 4

Ingredients:

- ½ cup chicken stock
- 1 cup fresh orange juice
- 1 tbsp. coconut oil
- 1 tbsp. tapioca starch
- 2 garlic cloves, minced
- 2 tbsp. fresh lemon juice
- 2 tsp. fresh rosemary, minced
- 2 tsp. orange zest
- 4 salmon fillets, skins removed
- Salt and pepper to taste

Directions:

1. Season the salmon fillet on both sides.

2. In a skillet, heat coconut oil over medium high heat. Cook the salmon fillets for 5 minutes on eac side. Set aside.
3. In a mixing bowl, combine the orange juice, chicken stock, lemon juice and orange zest.
4. In the skillet, sauté the garlic and rosemary for minutes and pour the orange juice mixture. Bring to a boil. Lower the heat to medium low and simmer. Season with salt and pepper to taste.
5. Pour the sauce all over the salmon fillet then serve.

Nutrition:

Calories: 493;

Fat: 17.9g;

Protein: 66.7g;

Carbs: 12.8g

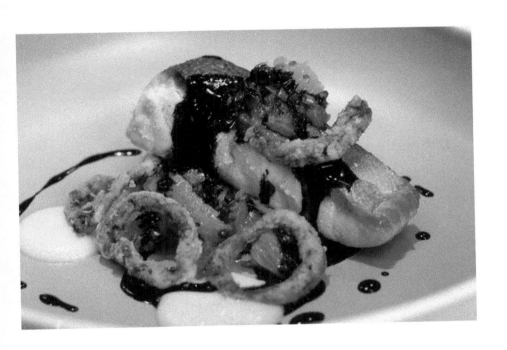

Orange Herbed Sauced White Bass

Preparation Time: 10 minutes

Cooking Time: 33 minutes

Servings: 6

Ingredients:

- ¼ cup thinly sliced green onions
- ½ cup orange juice
- 1 ½ tbsp. fresh lemon juice
- 1 ½ tbsp. olive oil
- 1 large onion, halved, thinly sliced
- 1 large orange, unpeeled, sliced
- 3 tbsp. chopped fresh dill
- 6 3-oz skinless white bass fillets
- Additional unpeeled orange slices

Directions:

1. Grease a 13 x 9-inch glass baking dish and preheat oven to 400oF.
2. Arrange orange slices in single layer on baking dish, top with onion slices, seasoned with pepper and salt plus drizzled with oil.
3. Pop in the oven and roast for 25 minutes or until onions are tender and browned.
4. Remove from oven and increased oven temperature to 450oF.
5. Push onion and orange slices on sides of dish and place bass fillets in middle of dish. Season with 1 ½ tbsp. dill, pepper and salt. Arrange onions and orange slices on top of fish and pop into the oven.
6. Roast for 8 minutes or until salmon is opaque and flaky.
7. In a small bowl, mix 1 ½ tbsp. dill, lemon juice, green onions and orange juice.
8. Transfer salmon to a serving plate, discard roasted onions, drizzle with the newly made orange sauce and garnish with fresh orange slices. Serve and enjoy.

Nutrition:

Calories: 312.42;

Protein: 84.22;

Fat: 23.14;

Carbs: 33.91g

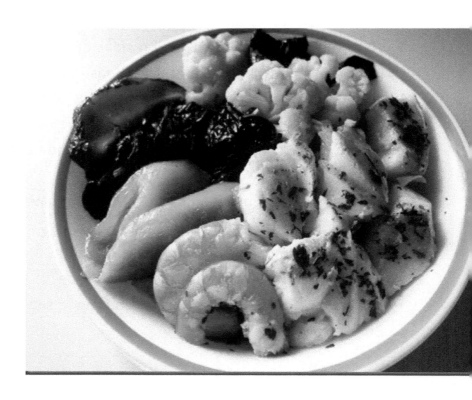

Pan Fried Tuna with Herbs and Nut

Preparation Time: 10 minutes

Cooking Time: 5 minutes

Servings: 4

Ingredients:

- ¼ cup almonds, chopped finely
- ¼ cup fresh tangerine juice
- ½ tsp. fennel seeds, chopped finely
- ½ tsp. ground pepper, divided
- ½ tsp. sea salt, divided
- 1 tbsp. olive oil
- 2 tbsp.. fresh mint, chopped finely
- 2 tbsp.. red onion, chopped finely
- 4 pieces of 6-oz Tuna steak cut in half

Directions:

1. Mix fennel seeds, olive oil, mint, onion, tangerine juice and almonds in small bowl. Season with ¼ each of pepper and salt.
2. Season fish with the remaining pepper and salt.
3. On medium high fire, place a large nonstick fry pan and grease with cooking spray.
4. Pan fry tuna until desired doneness is reached or for one minute per side.
5. Transfer cooked tuna in serving plate, drizzle with dressing and serve.

Nutrition:

Calories: 272;

Fat: 9.7 g;

Protein: 42 g;

Carbs: 4.2 g

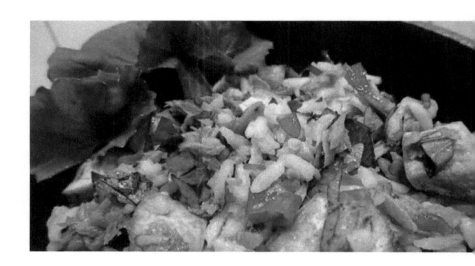

Paprika Salmon and Green Beans

Preparation Time: 10 minutes

Cooking Time: 20 minutes

Servings: 3

Ingredients:

- ¼ cup olive oil
- ½ tbsp. onion powder
- ½ tsp. bouillon powder
- ½ tsp. cayenne pepper
- 1 tbsp. smoked paprika
- 1-lb. green beans
- 2 tsp. minced garlic
- 3 tbsp. fresh herbs
- 6 oz. of salmon steak
- Salt and pepper to taste

Directions:

1. Preheat the oven to 400°F.

2. Grease a baking sheet and set aside.
3. Heat a skillet over medium low heat and add the olive oil. Sauté the garlic, smoked paprika, fresh herbs, cayenne pepper and onion powder. Stir for a minute then let the mixture sit for 5 minutes. Set aside.
4. Put the salmon steaks in a bowl and add salt and the paprika spice mixture. Rub to coat the salmon well.
5. Place the salmon on the baking sheet and cook for 18 minutes.
6. Meanwhile, blanch the green beans in boiling water with salt.
7. Serve the beans with the salmon.

Nutrition:

Calories: 945.8;

Fat: 66.6 g;

Protein: 43.5 g;

Carbs: 43.1 g

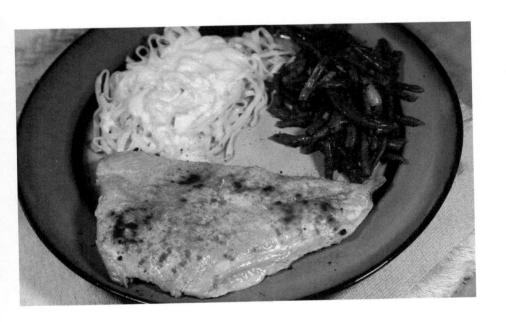

Pecan Crusted Trout

Preparation Time: 10 minutes

Cooking Time: 12 minutes

Servings: 4

Ingredients:

- ½ cup crushed pecans
- ½ tsp. grated fresh ginger
- 1 egg, beaten
- 1 tsp. crush dried rosemary
- 1 tsp. salt
- 4 4-oz trout fillets
- Black pepper to taste
- Cooking spray
- Whole wheat flour, as needed

Directions:

1. Grease baking sheet lightly with cooking spray and preheat oven to 400oF.

2. In a shallow bowl, combine black pepper, salt, rosemary and pecans. In another shallow bowl, add whole wheat flour. In a third bowl, add beaten egg.

3. To prepare fish, dip in flour until covered well. Shake off excess flour. Then dip into beaten egg until coated well. Let excess egg drip off before dipping trout fillet into pecan crumbs. Press the trout lightly onto pecan crumbs to make it stick to the fish.

4. Place breaded fish onto prepared pan. Repeat process for remaining fillets.

5. Pop into the oven and bake for 10 to 12 minutes or until fish is flaky.

Nutrition:

Calories: 329;

Fat: 19g;

Protein: 26.95g;

Carbs: 3g

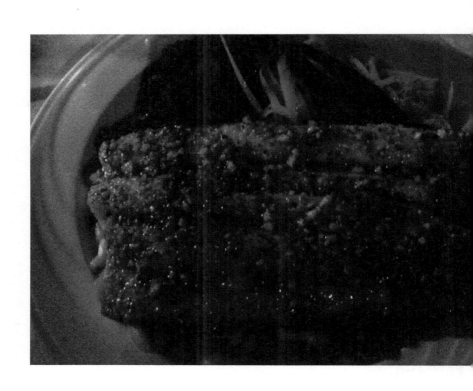

Pesto and Lemon Halibut

Preparation Time: 10 minutes

Cooking Time: 10 minutes

Servings: 4

Ingredients:

- 1 tbsp. fresh lemon juice
- 1 tbsp. lemon rind, grated
- 2 garlic cloves, peeled
- 2 tbsp. olive oil
- ¼ cup Parmesan Cheese, freshly grated
- 2/3 cups firmly packed basil leaves
- 1/8 tsp. freshly ground black pepper
- ¼ tsp. salt, divided
- 4 pcs 6-oz halibut fillets

Directions:

1. Preheat grill to medium fire and grease grate with cooking spray.
2. Season fillets with pepper and 1/8 tsp. salt. Place on grill and cook until halibut is flaky around 4 minutes per side.
3. Meanwhile, make your lemon pesto by combining lemon juice, lemon rind, garlic, olive oil, Parmesan cheese, basil leaves and remaining salt in a

blender. Pulse mixture until finely minced but not pureed.

4.   Once fish is done cooking, transfer to a serving platter, pour over the lemon pesto sauce, serve and enjoy.

Nutrition:

Calories: 277.4;

Fat: 13g;

Protein: 38.7g;

Carbs: 1.4g

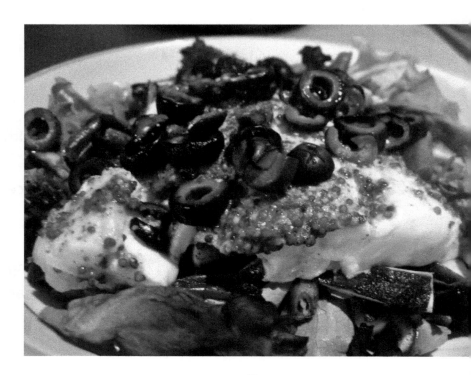

Red Peppers & Pineapple Topped Mahi-Mahi

Preparation Time: 10 minutes

Cooking Time: 30 minutes

Servings: 4

Ingredients:

- ¼ tsp. black pepper
- ¼ tsp. salt
- 1 cup whole wheat couscous
- 1 red bell pepper, diced
- 2 1/3 cups low sodium chicken broth
- 2 cups chopped fresh pineapple
- 2 tbsp.. chopped fresh chives
- 2 teaspoon. olive oil
- 4 pieces of skinless, boneless mahi mahi (dolphin fish) fillets (around 4-oz each)

Directions:

1. On high fire, add 1 1/3 cups broth to a small saucepan and heat until boiling. Once boiling, add couscous. Turn off fire, cover and set aside to allow liquid to be fully absorbed around 5 minutes
2. On medium high fire, place a large nonstick saucepan and heat oil.
3. Season fish on both sides with pepper and salt. Add mahi mahi to hot pan and pan fry until golden around one minute each side. Once cooked, transfer to plate.
4. On same pan, sauté bell pepper and pineapples until soft, around 2 minutes on medium high fire.
5. Add couscous to pan along with chives, and remaining broth.
6. On top of the mixture in pan, place fish. With foil cover pan and continue cooking until fish is steaming and tender underneath the foil, around 3-5 minutes.

Nutrition:

Calories: 302;

Protein: 43.1g;

Fat: 4.8g;

Carbs: 22.0g

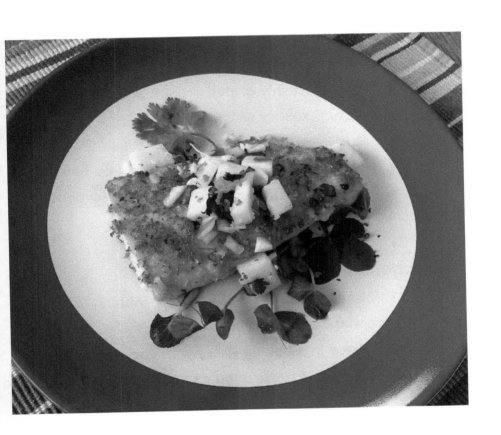

Roasted Halibut with Banana Relish

Preparation Time: 10 minutes

Cooking Time: 12 minutes

Servings: 4

Ingredients:

- ¼ cup cilantro
- ½ tsp. freshly grated orange zest
- ½ tsp. kosher salt, divided
- 1 lb. halibut or any deep-water fish
- 1 tsp. ground coriander, divided into half
- 2 oranges (peeled, segmented and chopped)
- 2 ripe bananas, diced
- 2 tbsp. lime juice

Directions:

1. In a pan, prepare the fish by rubbing ½ tsp. coriander and ¼ tsp. kosher salt.
2. Place in a baking sheet with cooking spray and bake for 8 to 12 minutes inside a 450°F preheate oven.
3. Prepare the relish by stirring the orange zest, bananas, chopped oranges, lime juice, cilantro an the rest of the salt and coriander in a medium bowl.
4. Spoon the relish over the roasted fish.
5. Serve and enjoy.

Nutrition:

Calories: 245.7;

Protein: 15.3g;

Fat: 6g;

Carbs: 21g

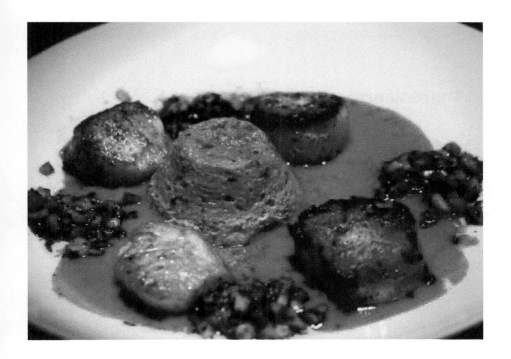

Roasted Pollock Fillet with Bacon and Leeks

Preparation Time: 10 minutes

Cooking Time: 30 minutes

Servings: 2

Ingredients:

- ¼ cup olive oil
- ½ cup white wine
- 1 ½ lbs. Pollock fillets
- 1 sprig fresh thyme
- 1 tbsp. chopped fresh thyme
- 2 tbsp.. olive oil
- 4 leeks, sliced

Directions:

1. Grease a 9x13 baking dish and preheat oven to 400°F F.
2. In baking pan add olive oil and leeks. Toss to combine.

3. Pop into the oven and roast for 10 minutes.

4. Remove from oven; add white wine and 1 tbsp. chopped thyme. Return to oven and roast for another 10 minutes.

5. Remove pan from oven and add fish on top. With a spoon, spoon olive oil mixture onto fish until coated fully. Return to oven and roast for another ten minutes.

6. Remove from oven, garnish with a sprig of thyme and serve.

Nutrition:

Calories: 442;

Carbs: 13.6 g;

Protein: 42.9 g;

Fat: 24 g

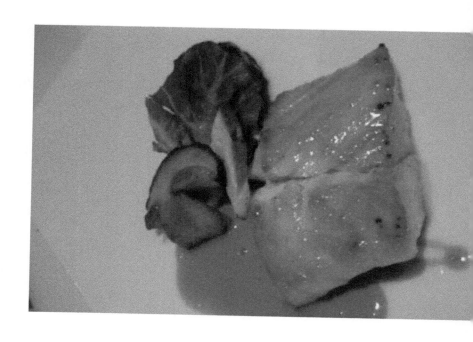

Scallops in Wine 'n Olive Oil

Preparation Time: 10 minutes

Cooking Time: 8 minutes

Servings: 4

Ingredients:

- ¼ tsp. salt
- ½ cup dry white wine
- 1 ½ lbs. large sea scallops
- 1 ½ tsp. chopped fresh tarragon
- 2 tbsp. olive oil
- Black pepper – optional

Directions:

1. On medium high fire, place a large nonstick fry pan and heat oil.
2. Add scallops and fry for 3 minutes per side or until edges are lightly browned. Transfer to a serving plate.
3. On same pan, add salt, tarragon and wine while scraping pan to loosen browned bits.
4. Turn off fire.
5. Pour sauce over scallops and serve.

Nutrition:

Calories: 205.2;

Fat: 8 g;

Protein: 28.6 g;

Carbs: 4.7 g

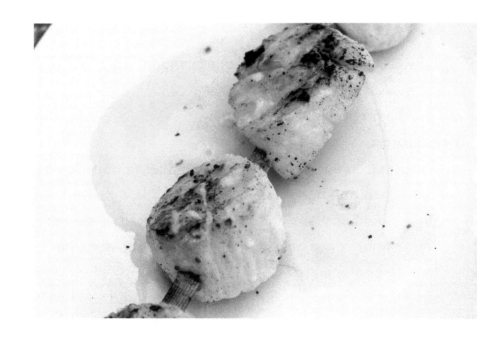

Seafood Stew Cioppino

Preparation Time: 10 minutes

Cooking Time: 40 minutes

Servings: 6

Ingredients:

- ¼ cup Italian parsley, chopped
- ¼ tsp. dried basil
- ¼ tsp. dried thyme
- ½ cup dry white wine like pinot grigio
- ½ lb. King crab legs, cut at each joint
- ½ onion, chopped
- ½ tsp. red pepper flakes (adjust to desired spiciness)
- 1 28-oz can crushed tomatoes
- 1 lb. mahi mahi, cut into ½-inch cubes
- 1 lb. raw shrimp
- 1 tbsp. olive oil
- 2 bay leaves
- 2 cups clam juice
- 50 live clams, washed
- 6 cloves garlic, minced
- Pepper and salt to taste

Directions:

1. On medium fire, place a stockpot and heat oil.
2. Add onion and for 4 minutes sauté until soft.

3. Add bay leaves, thyme, basil, red pepper flakes and garlic. Cook for a minute while stirring a bit.

4. Add clam juice and tomatoes. Once simmering, place fire to medium low and cook for 20 minutes uncovered.

5. Add white wine and clams. Cover and cook for 5 minutes or until clams have slightly opened.

6. Stir pot then add fish pieces, crab legs and shrimps. Do not stir soup to maintain the fish's shape. Cook while covered for 4 minutes or until clams are fully opened; fish and shrimps are opaque and cooked.

7. Season with pepper and salt to taste.

8. Transfer Cioppino to serving bowls and garnish with parsley before serving.

Nutrition:

Calories: 371;

Carbs: 15.5 g;

Protein: 62 g;

Fat: 6.8 g

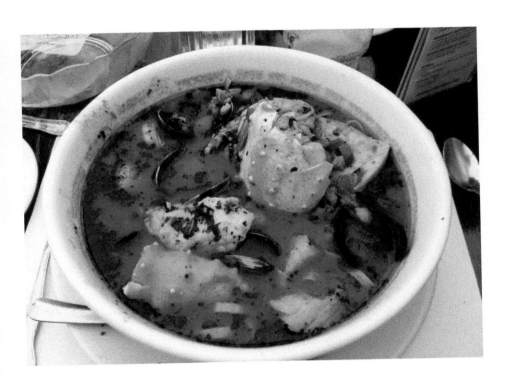

Simple Cod Piccata

Preparation Time: 10 minutes

Cooking Time: 15 minutes

Servings: 3

Ingredients:

- ¼ cup capers, drained
- ½ tsp. salt
- ¾ cup chicken stock
- 1/3 cup almond flour
- 1-lb. cod fillets, patted dry
- 2 tbsp. fresh parsley, chopped
- 2 tbsp. grapeseed oil
- 3 tbsp. extra-virgin oil
- 3 tbsp. lemon juice

Directions:

1. In a bowl, combine the almond flour and salt.
2. Dredge the fish in the almond flour to coat. Set aside.

3. Heat a little bit of olive oil to coat a large skillet. Heat the skillet over medium high heat. Add grapeseed oil. Cook the cod for 3 minutes on each side to brown. Remove from the plate and place on a paper towel-lined plate.
4. In a saucepan, mix together the chicken stock, capers and lemon juice. Simmer to reduce the sauce to half. Add the remaining grapeseed oil.
5. Drizzle the fried cod with the sauce and sprinkle with parsley.

Nutrition:

Calories: 277.1;

Fat: 28.3 g;

Protein: 21.9 g;

Carbs: 3.7 g

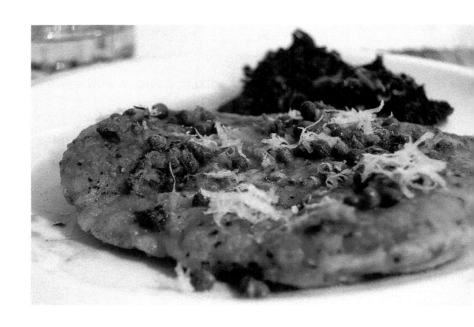

Smoked Trout Tartine

Preparation Time: 10 minutes

Cooking Time: 0 minutes

Servings: 4

Ingredients:

- ½ 15-oz can cannellini beans
- ½ cup diced roasted red peppers
- ¾ lb. smoked trout, flaked into bite-sized pieces
- 1 stalk celery, finely chopped
- 1 tbsp. extra virgin olive oil
- 1 tsp. chopped fresh dill
- 1 tsp. Dijon mustard
- 2 tbsp. capers, rinsed and drained
- 2 tbsp. freshly squeezed lemon juice
- 2 tsp. minced onion
- 4 large whole grain bread, toasted
- Dill sprigs – for garnish
- Pinch of sugar

Directions:

1. Mix sugar, mustard, olive oil and lemon juice in a big bowl.
2. Add the rest of the ingredients except for toasted bread.
3. Toss to mix well.
4. Evenly divide fish mixture on top of bread slices and garnish with dill sprigs.
5. Serve and enjoy.

Nutrition:

Calories: 348.1;

Protein: 28.2 g;

Fat: 10.1g;

Carbs: 36.1g

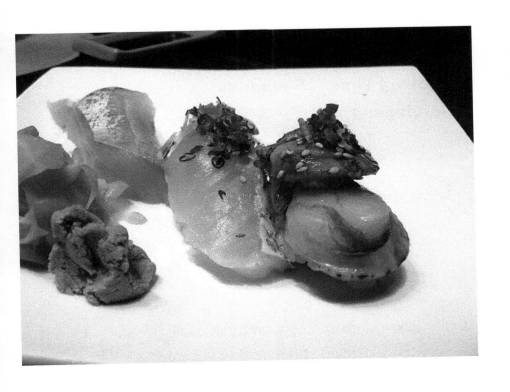

Steamed Mussels Thai Style

Preparation Time: 10 minutes

Cooking Time: 15 minutes

Servings: 4

Ingredients:

- ¼ cup minced shallots
- ½ tsp. Madras curry
- 1 cup dry white wine
- 1 small bay leaf
- 1 tbsp. chopped fresh basil
- 1 tbsp. chopped fresh cilantro
- 1 tbsp. chopped fresh mint
- 2 lbs. mussel, cleaned and debearded
- 2 tbsp. butter
- 4 medium garlic cloves, minced

Directions:

1. In a large heavy bottomed pot, on medium high fire add to pot the curry powder, bay leaf, wine plus the minced garlic and shallots. Bring to a boil and simmer for 3 minutes.
2. Add the cleaned mussels, stir, cover, and cook for 3 minutes.
3. Stir mussels again, cover, and cook for another 2 or 3 minutes. Cooking is done when majority of shells have opened.
4. With a slotted spoon, transfer cooked mussels in a large bowl. Discard any unopened mussels.
5. Continue heating pot with sauce. Add butter and the chopped herbs.
6. Season with pepper and salt to taste.
7. Once good, pour over mussels, serve and enjoy.

Nutrition:

Calories: 407.2;

Protein: 43.4g;

Fat: 21.2g;

Carbs: 10.8g

Tasty Tuna Scaloppine

Preparation Time: 10 minutes

Cooking Time: 10 minutes

Servings: 4

Ingredients:

- ¼ cup chopped almonds
- ¼ cup fresh tangerine juice
- ½ tsp. fennel seeds
- ½ tsp. ground black pepper, divided
- ½ tsp. salt
- 1 tbsp. extra virgin olive oil
- 2 tbsp. chopped fresh mint
- 2 tbsp. chopped red onion
- 4 6-oz sushi-grade Yellowfin tuna steaks, each split in half horizontally
- Cooking spray

Directions:

1. In a small bowl mix fennel seeds, olive oil, mint, onion, tangerine juice, almonds, ¼ tsp. pepper and ¼ tsp. salt. Combine thoroughly.
2. Season fish with remaining salt and pepper.
3. On medium high fire, place a large nonstick pan and grease with cooking spray. Pan fry fish in two batches cooking each side for a minute.
4. Fish is best served with a side of salad greens or a half cup of cooked brown rice.

Nutrition:

Calories: 405;

Protein: 27.5g;

Fat: 11.9g;

Carbs: 27.5

Thyme and Lemon on Baked Salmon

Preparation Time: 10 minutes

Cooking Time: 25 minutes

Servings: 2

Ingredients:

- 1 32-oz salmon fillet
- 1 lemon, sliced thinly
- 1 tbsp. capers
- 1 tbsp. fresh thyme
- Olive oil for drizzling
- Pepper and salt to taste

Directions:

1. In a foil line baking sheet, place a parchment paper on top.
2. Place salmon with skin side down on parchment paper.
3. Season generously with pepper and salt.
4. Place capers on top of fillet. Cover with thinly sliced lemon.
5. Garnish with thyme.
6. Pop in cold oven and bake for 25 minutes at 400°F settings.
7. Serve right away and enjoy.

Nutrition:

Calories: 684.4;

Protein: 94.3g;

Fat: 32.7g;

Carbs: 4.3g

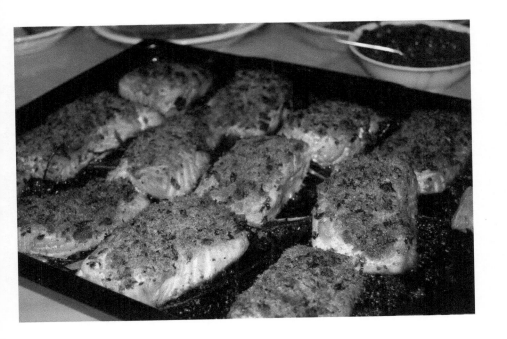

Warm Caper Tapenade on Cod

Preparation Time: 10 minutes

Cooking Time: 30 minutes

Servings: 4

Ingredients:

- ¼ cup chopped cured olives
- ¼ tsp. freshly ground pepper
- 1 ½ tsp. chopped fresh oregano
- 1 cup halved cherry tomatoes
- 1 lb. cod fillet
- 1 tbsp. capers, rinsed and chopped
- 1 tbsp. minced shallot
- 1 tsp. balsamic vinegar
- 3 tsp. extra virgin olive oil, divided

Directions:

1. Grease baking sheet with cooking spray and preheat oven to 450oF.

2. Place cod on prepared baking sheet. Rub with 2 tsp. oil and season with pepper.
3. Roast in oven for 15 to 20 minutes or until cod is flaky.
4. While waiting for cod to cook, on medium fire, place a small fry pan and heat 1 tsp. oil.
5. Sauté shallots for a minute.
6. Add tomatoes and cook for two minutes or until soft.
7. Add capers and olives. Sauté for another minute.
8. Add vinegar and oregano. Turn off fire and stir to mix well.
9. Evenly divide cod into 4 serving and place on a plate.
10. 1 To serve, top cod with Caper-Olive-Tomato Tapenade and enjoy.

Nutrition:

Calories: 107;

Fat: 2.9g;

Protein: 17.6g;

Carbs: 2.0g

Yummy Salmon Panzanella

Preparation Time: 10 minutes

Cooking Time: 10 minutes

Servings: 4

Ingredients:

- ¼ cup thinly sliced fresh basil
- ¼ cup thinly sliced red onion
- ¼ tsp. freshly ground pepper, divided
- ½ tsp. salt
- 1 lb. center cut salmon, skinned and cut into 4 equal portions
- 1 medium cucumber, peeled, seeded, and cut into 1-inch slices
- 1 tbsp. capers, rinsed and chopped
- 2 large tomatoes, cut into 1-inch pieces
- 2 thick slices day old whole grain bread, sliced into 1-inch cubes
- 3 tbsp. extra virgin olive oil
- 3 tbsp. red wine vinegar
- 8 Kalamata olives, pitted and chopped

Directions:

1. Grease grill grate and preheat grill to high.
2. In a large bowl, whisk 1/8 tsp. pepper, capers, vinegar, and olives. Add oil and whisk well.
3. Stir in basil, onion, cucumber, tomatoes, and bread.

68

4. Season both sides of salmon with remaining pepper and salt.
5. Grill on high for 4 minutes per side.
6. Into 4 plates, evenly divide salad, top with grilled salmon, and serve.

Nutrition:

Calories: 383;

Fat: 20.6g;

Protein: 34.8g;

Carbs: 13.6g

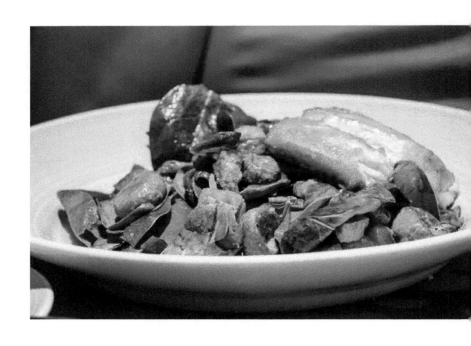

Fish and Orzo

Preparation Time: 10 minutes

Cooking Time: 35 minutes

Servings: 4

Ingredients:

- 1 tsp. garlic, minced
- 1 tsp. red pepper, crushed
- 2 shallots, chopped
- 1 tbsp. olive oil
- 1 tsp. anchovy paste
- 1 tbsp. oregano, chopped
- 2 tbsp. black olives, pitted and chopped
- 2 tbsp. capers, drained
- 15 oz. canned tomatoes, crushed
- A pinch of salt and black pepper
- 4 cod fillets, boneless
- 1 oz. feta cheese, crumbled
- 1 tbsp. parsley, chopped
- 3 cups chicken stock
- 1 cup orzo pasta
- Zest of 1 lemon, grated

Directions:

1. Heat up a pan with the oil over medium heat, add the garlic, red pepper and the shallots and sauté for 5 minutes.
2. Add the anchovy paste, oregano, black olives, capers, tomatoes, salt and pepper, stir and cook for 5 minutes more.
3. Add the cod fillets, sprinkle the cheese and the parsley on top, introduce in the oven and bake at 375°F for 15 minutes more.
4. Meanwhile, put the stock in a pot, bring to a boil over medium heat, add the orzo and the lemon zest, bring to a simmer, cook for 10 minutes, fluff with a fork, and divide between plates.
5. Top each serving with the fish mix and serve.

Nutrition: Calories 402, Fat 21g, Fiber 8g, Carbs 21g, Protein 31g

Baked Sea Bass

Preparation Time: 10 minutes

Cooking Time: 12 minutes

Servings: 4

Ingredients:

- 4 sea bass fillets, boneless
- Sal and black pepper to the taste
- 2 cups potato chips, crushed
- 1 tbsp. mayonnaise

Directions:

1. Season the fish fillets with salt and pepper, brush with the mayonnaise and dredge each in the potato chips.
2. Arrange the fillets on a baking sheet lined with parchment paper and bake at 400°F for 12 minutes.
3. Divide the fish between plates and serve with a side salad.

Nutrition: Calories 228, Fat 8.6g, Fiber 0.6g, Carbs 9.3g, Protein 25g

Fish and Tomato Sauce

Preparation Time: 10 minutes

Cooking Time: 30 minutes

Servings: 4

Ingredients:

- 4 cod fillets, boneless
- 2 garlic cloves, minced
- 2 cups cherry tomatoes, halved
- 1 cup chicken stock
- A pinch of salt and black pepper
- ¼ cup basil, chopped

Directions:

1. Put the tomatoes, garlic, salt and pepper in a pan, heat up over medium heat and cook for 5 minutes.
2. Add the fish and the rest of the ingredients, brin to a simmer, cover the pan and cook for 25 minutes.
3. Divide the mix between plates and serve.

Nutrition: Calories 180, Fat 1.9g, Fiber 1.4g, Carbs 5.3g, Protein 33.8g

Halibut and Quinoa Mix

Preparation Time: 10 minutes

Cooking Time: 12 minutes

Servings: 4

Ingredients:

- 4 halibut fillets, boneless
- 2 tbsp. olive oil
- 1 tsp. rosemary, dried
- 2 tsp. cumin, ground
- 1 tbsp. coriander, ground
- 2 tsp. cinnamon powder
- 2 tsp. oregano, dried
- A pinch of salt and black pepper
- 2 cups quinoa, cooked
- 1 cup cherry tomatoes, halved
- 1 avocado, peeled, pitted and sliced
- 1 cucumber, cubed
- ½ cup black olives, pitted and sliced

- Juice of 1 lemon

Directions:

1. In a bowl, combine the fish with the rosemary, cumin, coriander, cinnamon, oregano, salt and pepper and toss.
2. Heat up a pan with the oil over medium heat, add the fish, and sear for 2 minutes on each side.
3. Introduce the pan in the oven and bake the fish at 425°F for 7 minutes.
4. Meanwhile, in a bowl, mix the quinoa with the remaining ingredients, toss and divide between plates.
5. Add the fish next to the quinoa mix and serve right away.

Nutrition: Calories 364, Fat 15.4g, Fiber 11.2g, Carbs 56.4g, Protein 24.5g

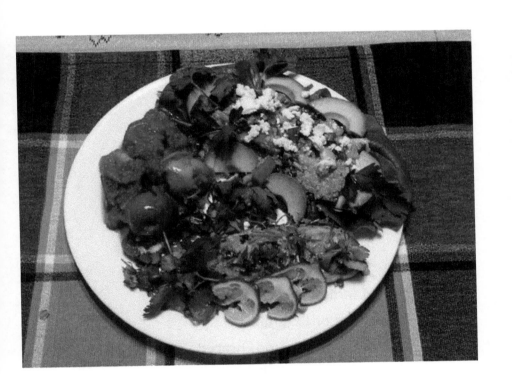

Lemon and Dates Barramundi

Preparation Time: 10 minutes

Cooking Time: 12 minutes

Servings: 2

Ingredients:

- 2 barramundi fillets, boneless
- 1 shallot, sliced
- 4 lemon slices
- Juice of ½ lemon
- Zest of 1 lemon, grated
- 2 tbsp. olive oil
- 6 oz. baby spinach
- ¼ cup almonds, chopped
- 4 dates, pitted and chopped
- ¼ cup parsley, chopped
- Salt and black pepper to the taste

Directions:

1. Season the fish with salt and pepper and arrange on 2 parchment paper pieces.
2. Top the fish with the lemon slices, drizzle the lemon juice, and then top with the other ingredients except the oil.
3. Drizzle 1 tbsp. oil over each fish mix, wrap the parchment paper around the fish shaping to packets and arrange them on a baking sheet.
4. Bake at 400°F for 12 minutes, cool the mix a bit, unfold, divide everything between plates and serve.

Nutrition: Calories 232, Fat 16.5g, Fiber 11.1g, Carbs 24.8g, Protein 6.5g

Fish Cakes

Preparation Time: 10 minutes

Cooking Time: 10 minutes

Servings: 6

Ingredients:

- 20 oz. canned sardines, drained and mashed we
- 2 garlic cloves, minced
- 2 tbsp. dill, chopped
- 1 yellow onion, chopped
- 1 cup panko breadcrumbs
- 1 egg, whisked
- A pinch of salt and black pepper
- 2 tbsp. lemon juice
- 5 tbsp. olive oil

Directions:

1. In a bowl, combine the sardines with the garlic, dill and the rest of the ingredients except the oil, stir well and shape medium cakes out of this mix.
2. Heat up a pan with the oil over medium-high heat, add the fish cakes, cook for 5 minutes on each side.
3. Serve the cakes with a side salad.

Nutrition: Calories 288, Fat 12.8g, Fiber 10.2g, Carbs 22.2g, Protein 6.8g

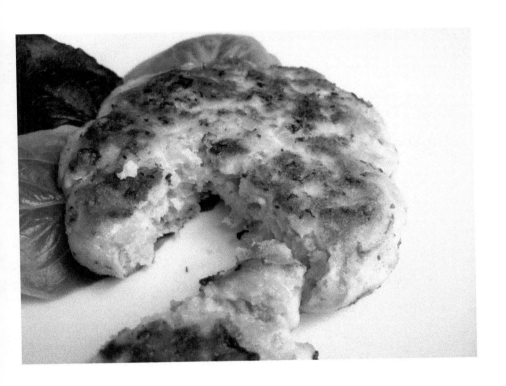

81

Catfish Fillets and Rice

Preparation Time: 10 minutes

Cooking Time: 55 minutes

Servings: 2

Ingredients:

- 2 catfish fillets, boneless
- 2 tbsp. Italian seasoning
- 2 tbsp. olive oil
- For the rice:
- 1 cup brown rice
- 2 tbsp. olive oil
- 1 and ½ cups water
- ½ cup green bell pepper, chopped
- 2 garlic cloves, minced
- ½ cup white onion, chopped
- 2 tsp. Cajun seasoning
- ½ tsp. garlic powder
- Salt and black pepper to the taste

Directions:

1. Heat up a pot with 2 tbsp. oil over medium heat, add the onion, garlic, garlic powder, salt and pepper and sauté for 5 minutes.
2. Add the rice, water, bell pepper and the seasoning, bring to a simmer and cook over medium heat for 40 minutes.
3. Heat up a pan with 2 tbsp. oil over medium heat, add the fish and the Italian seasoning, and cook for 5 minutes on each side.
4. Divide the rice between plates, add the fish on top and serve.

Nutrition: Calories 261, Fat 17.6g, Fiber 12.2g, Carbs 24.8g, Protein 12.5g

Halibut Pan

Preparation Time: 10 minutes

Cooking Time: 20 minutes

Servings: 4

Ingredients:

- 4 halibut fillets, boneless
- 1 red bell pepper, chopped
- 2 tbsp. olive oil
- 1 yellow onion, chopped
- 4 garlic cloves, minced
- ½ cup chicken stock
- 1 tsp. basil, dried
- ½ cup cherry tomatoes, halved
- 1/3 cup kalamata olives, pitted and halved
- Salt and black pepper to the taste

Directions:

1. Heat up a pan with the oil over medium heat, add the fish, cook for 5 minutes on each side and divide between plates.
2. Add the onion, bell pepper, garlic and tomatoes to the pan, stir and sauté for 3 minutes.
3. Add salt, pepper and the rest of the ingredients, toss, cook for 3 minutes more, divide next to the fish and serve.

Nutrition: Calories 253, Fat 8g, Fiber 1g, Carbs 5g, Protein 28g

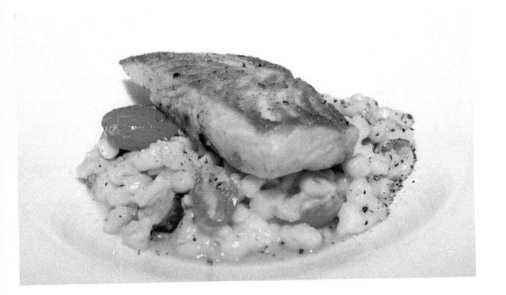

Baked Shrimp Mix

Preparation Time: 10 minutes

Cooking Time: 32 minutes

Servings: 4

Ingredients:

- 4 gold potatoes, peeled and sliced
- 2 fennel bulbs, trimmed and cut into wedges
- 2 shallots, chopped
- 2 garlic cloves, minced
- 3 tbsp. olive oil
- ½ cup kalamata olives, pitted and halved
- 2 lb. shrimp, peeled and deveined
- 1 tsp. lemon zest, grated
- 2 tsp. oregano, dried
- 4 oz. feta cheese, crumbled
- 2 tbsp. parsley, chopped

Directions:

1. In a roasting pan, combine the potatoes with 2 tbsp. oil, garlic and the rest of the ingredients except the shrimp, toss, introduce in the oven and bake at 450°F for 25 minutes.
2. Add the shrimp, toss, bake for 7 minutes more, divide between plates and serve.

Nutrition: Calories 341, Fat 19g, Fiber 9g, Carbs 34g, Protein 10g

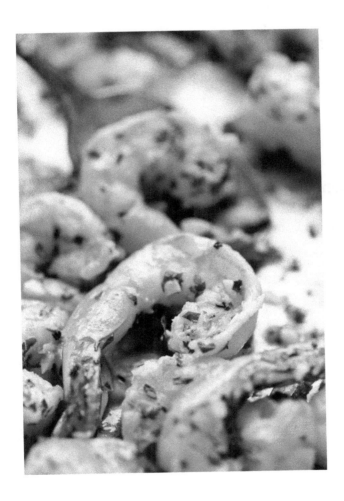

Shrimp and Lemon Sauce

Preparation Time: 10 minutes

Cooking Time: 15 minutes

Servings: 4

Ingredients:

- 1 lb. shrimp, peeled and deveined
- 1/3 cup lemon juice
- 4 egg yolks
- 2 tbsp. olive oil
- 1 cup chicken stock
- Salt and black pepper to the taste
- 1 cup black olives, pitted and halved
- 1 tbsp. thyme, chopped

Directions:

1. In a bowl, mix the lemon juice with the egg yolks and whisk well.

2. Heat up a pan with the oil over medium heat, add the shrimp and cook for 2 minutes on each side and transfer to a plate.
3. Heat up a pan with the stock over medium heat, add some of this over the egg yolks and lemon juice mix and whisk well.
4. Add this over the rest of the stock, also add salt and pepper, whisk well and simmer for 2 minutes.
5. Add the shrimp and the rest of the ingredients, toss and serve right away.

Nutrition: Calories 237, Fat 15.3g, Fiber 4.6g, Carbs 15.4g, Protein 7.6g

Shrimp and Beans Salad

Preparation Time: 10 minutes

Cooking Time: 4 minutes

Servings: 4

Ingredients:

- 1 lb. shrimp, peeled and deveined
- 30 oz. canned cannellini beans, drained and rinsed
- 2 tbsp. olive oil
- 1 cup cherry tomatoes, halved
- 1 tsp. lemon zest, grated
- ½ cup red onion, chopped
- 4 handfuls baby arugula
- A pinch of salt and black pepper
- For the dressing:
- 3 tbsp. red wine vinegar
- 2 garlic cloves, minced
- ½ cup olive oil

Directions:

1. Heat up a pan with 2 tbsp. oil over medium-high heat, add the shrimp and cook for 2 minutes on each side.
2. In a salad bowl, combine the shrimp with the beans and the rest of the ingredients except the ones for the dressing and toss.
3. In a separate bowl, combine the vinegar with ½ cup oil and the garlic and whisk well.
4. Pour over the salad, toss and serve right away.

Nutrition: Calories 207, Fat 12.3g, Fiber 6.6g, Carbs 15.4g, Protein 8.7g

Pecan Salmon Fillets

Preparation Time: 10 minutes

Cooking Time: 15 minutes

Servings: 6

Ingredients:

- 3 tbsp. olive oil
- 3 tbsp. mustard
- 5 tsp. honey
- 1 cup pecans, chopped
- 6 salmon fillets, boneless
- 1 tbsp. lemon juice
- 3 tsp. parsley, chopped
- Salt and pepper to the taste

Directions:

1. In a bowl, mix the oil with the mustard and honey and whisk well.
2. Put the pecans and the parsley in another bowl.
3. Season the salmon fillets with salt and pepper, arrange them on a baking sheet lined with parchment paper, brush with the honey and mustard mix and top with the pecans mix.
4. Introduce in the oven at 400°F, bake for 15 minutes, divide between plates, drizzle the lemon juice on top and serve.

Nutrition: Calories 282, Fat 15.5g, Fiber 8.5g, Carbs 20.9g, Protein 16.8g

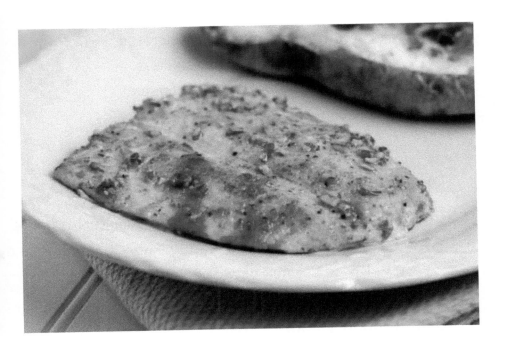

Salmon and Broccoli

Preparation Time: 10 minutes

Cooking Time: 20 minutes

Servings: 4

Ingredients:

- 2 tbsp. balsamic vinegar
- 1 broccoli head, florets separated
- 4 pieces salmon fillets, skinless
- 1 big red onion, roughly chopped
- 1 tbsp. olive oil
- Sea salt and black pepper to the taste

Directions:

1. In a baking dish, combine the salmon with the broccoli and the rest of the ingredients, introduce in the oven and bake at 390°F for 20 minutes.
2. Divide the mix between plates and serve.

Nutrition: Calories 302, Fat 15.5g, Fiber 8.5g, Carbs 18.9g, Protein 19.8g

Salmon and Peach Pan

Preparation Time: 10 minutes

Cooking Time: 11 minutes

Servings: 4

Ingredients:

- 1 tbsp. balsamic vinegar
- 1 tsp. thyme, chopped
- 1 tbsp. ginger, grated
- 2 tbsp. olive oil
- Sea salt and black pepper to the taste
- 3 peaches, cut into medium wedges
- 4 salmon fillets, boneless

Directions:

1. Heat up a pan with the oil over medium-high heat, add the salmon and cook for 3 minutes on each side.
2. Add the vinegar, the peaches and the rest of the ingredients, cook for 5 minutes more, divide everything between plates and serve.

Nutrition: Calories 293, Fat 17.1g, Fiber 4.1g, Carbs 26.4g, Protein 24.5g

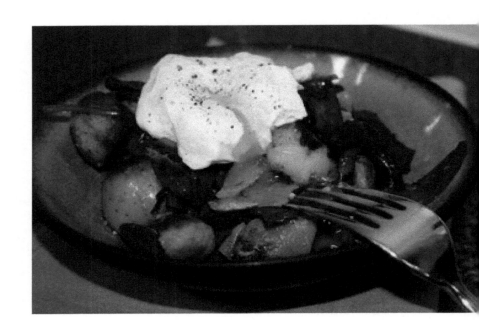

Tarragon Cod Fillets

Preparation Time: 10 minutes

Cooking Time: 12 minutes

Servings: 4

Ingredients:

- 4 cod fillets, boneless
- ¼ cup capers, drained
- 1 tbsp. tarragon, chopped
- Sea salt and black pepper to the taste
- 2 tbsp. olive oil
- 2 tbsp. parsley, chopped
- 1 tbsp. olive oil
- 1 tbsp. lemon juice

Directions:

1. Heat up a pan with the oil over medium-high heat, add the fish and cook for 3 minutes on each side.
2. Add the rest of the ingredients, cook everything for 7 minutes more, divide between plates and serve.

Nutrition: Calories 162, Fat 9.6g, Fiber 4.3g, Carbs 12.4g, Protein 16.5g

Salmon and Radish Mix

Preparation Time: 10 minutes

Cooking Time: 15 minutes

Servings: 4

Ingredients:

- 2 tbsp. olive oil
- 1 tbsp. balsamic vinegar
- 1 and ½ cup chicken stock
- 4 salmon fillets, boneless
- 2 garlic cloves, minced
- 1 tbsp. ginger, grated
- 1 cup radishes, grated
- ¼ cup scallions, chopped

Directions:

1. Heat up a pan with the oil over medium-high heat, add the salmon, cook for 4 minutes on each side and divide between plates
2. Add the vinegar and the rest of the ingredients t the pan, toss gently, cook for 10 minutes, add over the salmon and serve.

Nutrition: Calories 274, Fat 14.5g, Fiber 3.5g, Carbs 8.5g, Protein 22.3g

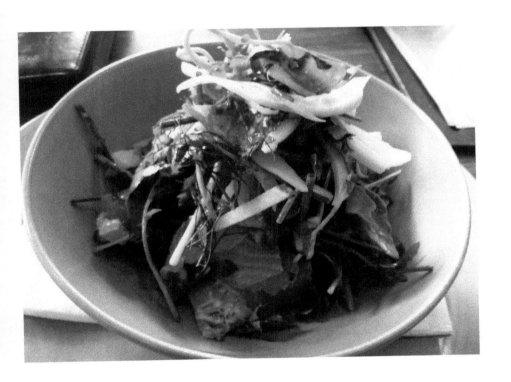

Smoked Salmon and Watercress Salad

Preparation Time: 5 minutes

Cooking Time: 0 minutes

Servings: 4

Ingredients:

- 2 bunches watercress
- 1 lb. smoked salmon, skinless, boneless and flaked
- 2 tsp. mustard
- ¼ cup lemon juice
- ½ cup Greek yogurt
- Salt and black pepper to the taste
- 1 big cucumber, sliced
- 2 tbsp. chives, chopped

Directions:

1. In a salad bowl, combine the salmon with the watercress and the rest of the ingredients toss an serve right away.

Nutrition: Calories 244, Fat 16.7g, Fiber 4.5g, Carbs 22.5g, Protein 15.6g

Salmon and Corn Salad

Preparation Time: 5 minutes

Cooking Time: 0 minutes

Servings: 4

Ingredients:

- ½ cup pecans, chopped
- 2 cups baby arugula
- 1 cup corn
- ¼ lb. smoked salmon, skinless, boneless and cut into small chunks
- 2 tbsp. olive oil
- 2 tbsp. lemon juice
- Sea salt and black pepper to the taste

Directions:

1. In a salad bowl, combine the salmon with the corn and the rest of the ingredients, toss and serve right away.

Nutrition: Calories 284, Fat 18.4g, Fiber 5.4g, Carbs 22.6g, Protein 17.4g

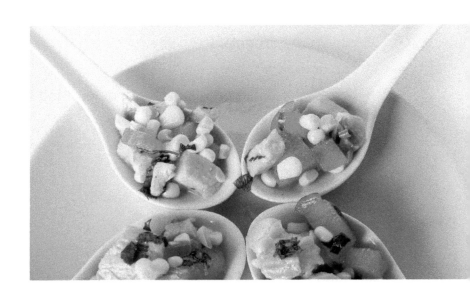

Cod and Mushrooms Mix

Preparation Time: 10 minutes

Cooking Time: 25 minutes

Servings: 4

Ingredients:

- 2 cod fillets, boneless
- 4 tbsp. olive oil
- 4 oz. mushrooms, sliced
- Sea salt and black pepper to the taste
- 12 cherry tomatoes, halved
- 8 oz. lettuce leaves, torn
- 1 avocado, pitted, peeled and cubed
- 1 red chili pepper, chopped
- 1 tbsp. cilantro, chopped
- 2 tbsp. balsamic vinegar
- 1 oz. feta cheese, crumbled

Directions:

1. Put the fish in a roasting pan, brush it with 2 tbsp. oil, sprinkle salt and pepper all over and bro under medium-high heat for 15 minutes. Meanwhile, heat up a pan with the rest of the oil over medium heat, add the mushrooms, stir and sauté for 5 minutes.
2. Add the rest of the ingredients, toss, cook for 5 minutes more and divide between plates.
3. Top with the fish and serve right away.

Nutrition: Calories 257, Fat 10g, Fiber 3.1g, Carbs 24.3g, Protein 19.4g

Sesame Shrimp Mix

Preparation Time: 10 minutes

Cooking Time: 0 minutes

Servings: 4

Ingredients:

- 2 tbsp. lime juice
- 3 tbsp. teriyaki sauce
- 2 tbsp. olive oil
- 8 cups baby spinach
- 14 oz. shrimp, cooked, peeled and deveined
- 1 cup cucumber, sliced
- 1 cup radish, sliced
- ¼ cup cilantro, chopped
- 2 tsp. sesame seeds, toasted

Directions:

1. In a bowl, mix the shrimp with the lime juice, spinach and the rest of the ingredients, toss and serve cold.

Nutrition: Calories 177, Fat 9g, Fiber 7.1g, Carbs 14.3g, Protein 9.4g

Creamy Curry Salmon

Preparation Time: 10 minutes

Cooking Time: 20 minutes

Servings: 2

Ingredients:

- 2 salmon fillets, boneless and cubed
- 1 tbsp. olive oil
- 1 tbsp. basil, chopped
- Sea salt and black pepper to the taste
- 1 cup Greek yogurt
- 2 tsp. curry powder
- 1 garlic clove, minced
- ½ tsp. mint, chopped

Directions:

1. Heat up a pan with the oil over medium-high heat, add the salmon and cook for 3 minutes.
2. Add the rest of the ingredients, toss, cook for 15 minutes more, divide between plates and serve.

Nutrition: Calories 284, Fat 14.1g, Fiber 8.5g, Carbs 26.7g, Protein 31.4g

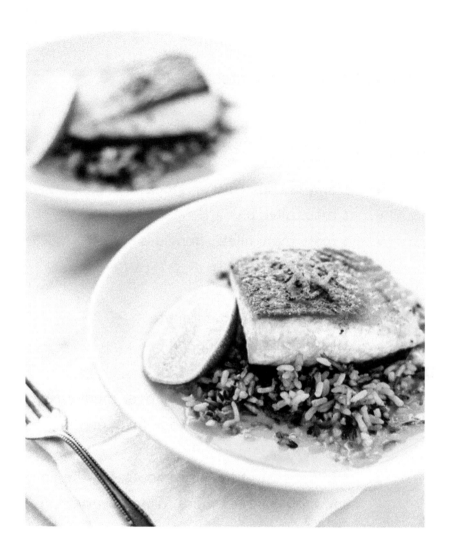

Mahi Mahi and Pomegranate Sauce

Preparation Time: 10 minutes

Cooking Time: 10 minutes

Servings: 4

Ingredients:

- 1 and ½ cups chicken stock
- 1 tbsp. olive oil
- 4 mahi mahi fillets, boneless
- 4 tbsp. tahini paste
- Juice of 1 lime
- Seeds from 1 pomegranate
- 1 tbsp. parsley, chopped

Directions:

1. Heat up a pan with the oil over medium-high heat, add the fish and cook for 3 minutes on each side.
2. Add the rest of the ingredients, flip the fish again cook for 4 minutes more, divide everything between plates and serve.

Nutrition: Calories 224, Fat 11.1g, Fiber 5.5g, Carbs 16.7g, Protein 11.4g

Smoked Salmon and Veggies Mix

Preparation Time: 10 minutes

Cooking Time: 20 minutes

Servings: 4

Ingredients:

- 3 red onions, cut into wedges
- ¾ cup green olives, pitted and halved
- 3 red bell peppers, roughly chopped
- ½ tsp. smoked paprika
- Salt and black pepper to the taste
- 3 tbsp. olive oil
- 4 salmon fillets, skinless and boneless
- 2 tbsp. chives, chopped

Directions:

1. In a roasting pan, combine the salmon with the onions and the rest of the ingredients, introduce in the oven and bake at 390°F for 20 minutes.
2. Divide the mix between plates and serve.

Nutrition: Calories 301, Fat 5.9g, Fiber 11.9g, Carbs 26.4g, Protein 22.4g

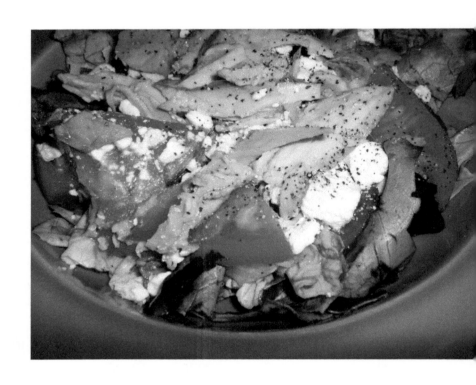

Lightning Source UK Ltd.
Milton Keynes UK
UKHW020651210521
384114UK00001B/76